A guide for people with

HEART FAILURE

by

Julia Ann Purcell, RN, MN, FAAN

Barbara J. Fletcher, RN, MN, FAAN

Over 5 million Americans have chronic heart failure. This book can help you and your loved ones understand and manage heart failure...living a longer, fuller life. You will learn how to:

> take the medications exactly as prescribed

> weigh daily for fluid buildup

> avoid excessive sodium intake

> balance exercise and rest

> make less work for your heart by not smoking and getting rid of excess weight

> control things like high blood pressure, diabetes, obesity, sleep apnea

This book offers guidelines that can help your heart work better. The book should not replace your doctor's advice or treatment.

Contents

® Order this book from :

PRITCHETT & HULL ASSOCIATES, INC.
3440 OAKCLIFF RD NE STE 126
ATLANTA GA 30340-3006

or call toll free: 800-241-4925

Copyright© 1989, 1993, 1995, 1999, 2004,
2006, 2010, 2012, 2016

This book is only to help you
learn, and should not be used
to replace any of your doctor's
advice or treatment.

Published and distributed by:
Pritchett & Hull Associates, Inc.

Printed in the U.S.A.

Heart Failure

A healthy heart pumps out enough oxygen-rich blood to feed all parts of the body. It should fully relax to fill up again with the incoming blood. Heart failure occurs when there are problems with either pumping and/or filling. Symptoms like shortness of breath, swelling in the belly, hands, legs and feet are common.

Heart failure can range from mild (more common) to severe. There are many factors involved:

> the cause of your heart problem

> the way your heart pumps and fills

> how your body reacts to it

> any extra demands on your heart, like being overweight or having high blood pressure

Most often, heart failure can be controlled with medicines, diet, rest and low-level exercise. Your heart failure symptoms may come and go or, in a few cases, go away completely.

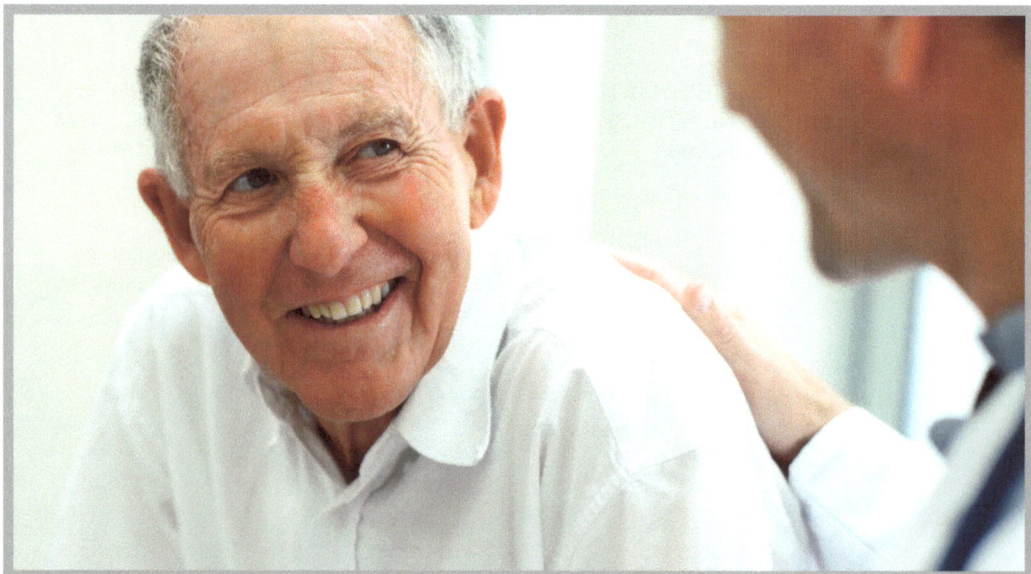

How you may feel

As heart failure gets worse, you may notice some or all of these:

- [ ] **sudden weight gain** (3–4 lbs in 1 to 2 days or 2 lbs overnight)

- [ ] **swelling of the legs and ankles**

- [ ] **swelling, bloating** (you feel full much earlier at meals) **or pain in the belly**

- [ ] **trouble sleeping unless propped up on 2 or more pillows** (can be caused by problems other than heart failure)

- [ ] **shortness of breath** (all of the time, with exertion or when waking up breathless at night)

- [ ] **frequent, dry, hacking cough** (most often when lying down)

- [ ] **loss of appetite** (or nausea)

You may also get tired from very little effort. This happens when blood flow is sluggish. You may wake up feeling tired or get drowsy in the afternoon. This is even more likely if you are not breathing well when you sleep. Your family may notice snoring or louder snoring than before.

Many of these symptoms can occur with problems other than heart failure. Your doctor or nurse will check your heart and lungs. Blood tests (and/or a sleep study) may help find out what is wrong.

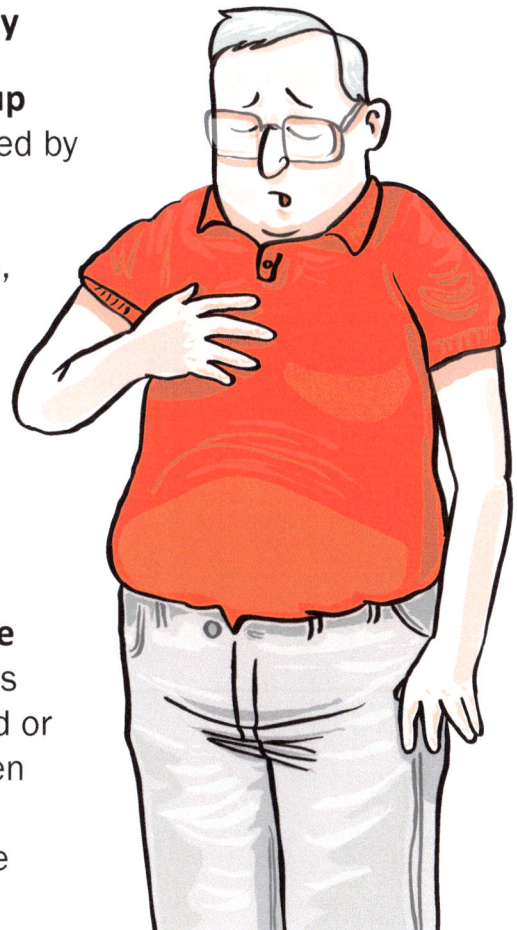

Blood returns from the veins to the **right** side of your heart. It is then pumped to your lungs to pick up oxygen on its way to the **left side of your heart.** The **left** heart pumps the blood out to your body arteries through the main artery (aorta).

If your heart failure is due to pumping weakness, it may start in the **right** or **left** side of your heart. But soon **both** left and right sides are strained.

right heart failure

When the right side of your heart has a pumping problem, blood backs up in your veins. You may not notice it, since veins can stretch and hold the extra blood.

Days or maybe weeks later, you may notice that your legs and ankles are swollen. You may also feel sore or swollen in the upper right side of your belly. And you may feel tired and not want to eat.

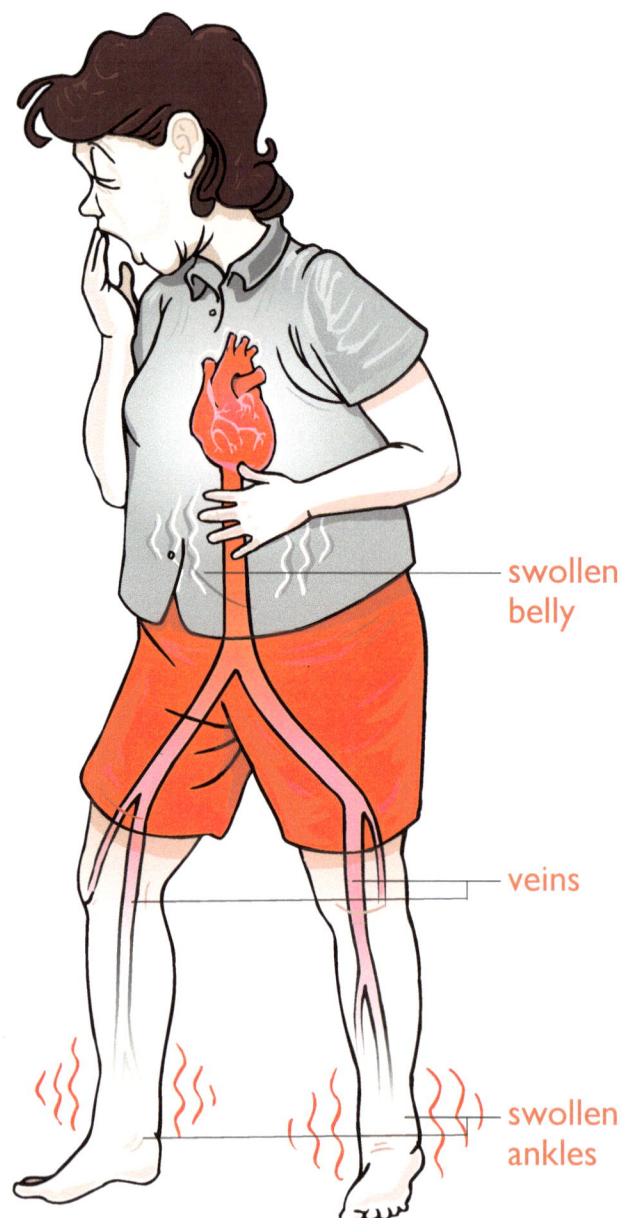

swollen belly

veins

swollen ankles

left heart failure

When the left side of your heart does not pump out all the blood it gets, fluid backs up into your lungs. You may:

> feel short of breath

> have trouble sleeping if you do not prop up on pillows

> wake up feeling out of breath

> have a dry hacking cough

You may also feel swollen or bloated. This is because your body is holding too much fluid. This adds to your heart's workload. Your weak heart has to pump all of this extra fluid along with the blood.

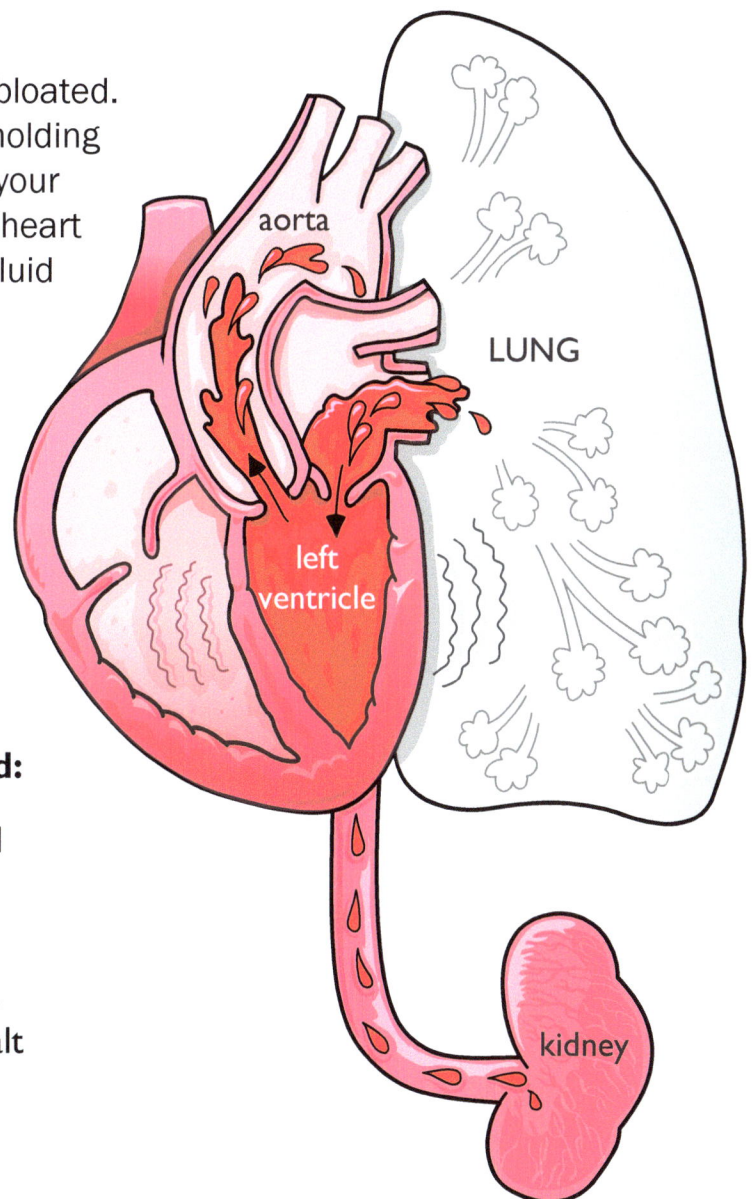

Why your body holds fluid:

A weak heart sends less blood to the kidneys. The kidneys think the body doesn't have enough blood. So, instead of passing out as much urine, the kidneys keep this water and salt in the blood. This adds more blood for the heart to pump.

aorta

LUNG

left ventricle

kidney

A sudden weight gain is one sign the kidneys are holding salt and water in your body. To check for this, **weigh each morning** after you urinate and before eating or getting dressed. **Write down your weight.**

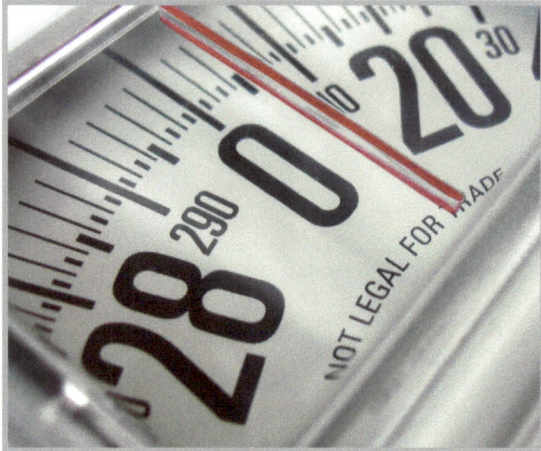

> Each time you weigh, make sure your scale is set on a hard surface (not carpet) and adjusted to zero.

> When checking your weight, think about how well you are eating. If you are eating less and losing pounds, you may not notice a gain from fluid.

> If you gain 3–4 lbs in 1 to 2 days of normal eating (or 2 lbs overnight), it is more likely due to fluid rather than food. Call your doctor or nurse for advice to get rid of this extra fluid before it weakens your heart more. Often, you need more diuretic ("water pill").

> Always write down your weight and any diuretics taken in a notebook lined off like this:

Date	Weight	Diuretic Taken

Heart Failure Testing

Your healthcare provider will order an EKG and one or more of these tests to detect, monitor and/or choose the best treatment for you. Often these treatments make you feel better and improve how your heart works.

Doppler echocardiogram (ECHO)

An echocardiogram is an ultrasound of your heart. Sound waves (sonography) are moved over the heart to show:

> problems with the heart muscle

> how well it pumps and relaxes

> the condition of your heart valves and the sac around the heart

A technician moves a hand-held scanner over your chest, taking pictures and recording them. You may feel some pressure as the scanner is pressed against your chest. Pictures can be made from several angles (two or three dimensional ECHO). These pictures show how the blood moves inside your heart and back and forth across your heart valves.

An echocardiogram also measures the heart's ejection fraction ("EF"). A normal EF is 50% or more.

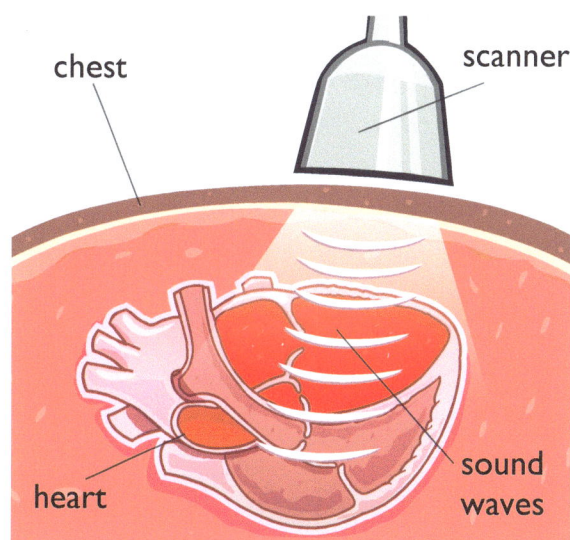

chest

scanner

heart

sound waves

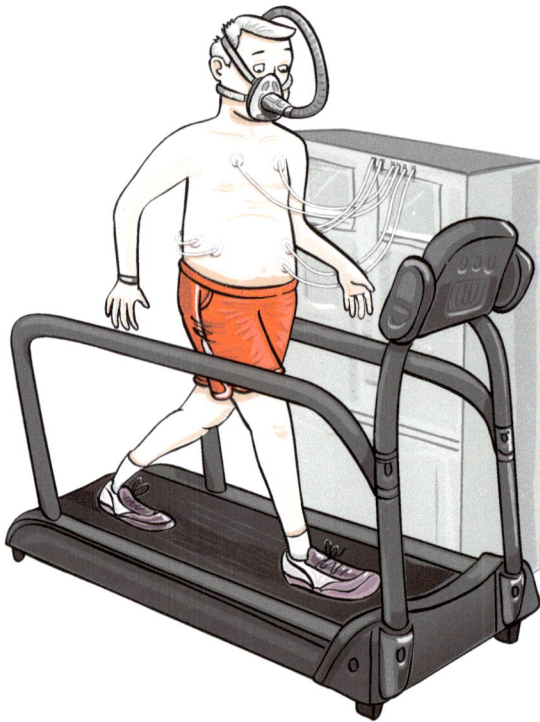

exercise test

This test records your heartbeat, EKG and blood pressure at rest, during exercise and just after exercise. You may be asked to walk on a treadmill or ride a stationary bike.

As you exercise, your workload is slowly increased to see how your heart responds. You may also be asked to breathe through a tube or mask to measure how much oxygen your body uses.

other tests are sometimes needed

A **cardiac catheterization** (heart cath) may be done to see if you have narrowing in your heart arteries. **Ultrafast CT* scans** can detect build-up of calcium in the heart arteries. **Multi-slice cardiac CT scans** take X-ray pictures of the heart, blood vessels, lungs and sac around the heart. Sometimes a "dye" is given (contrast) and pictures are made of the heart arteries.

Magnetic resonance imaging **(MRI)** may be needed to find the reason for heart failure. MRI offers more detail about the lower heart chambers. In some cases, an MRI is helpful to find out more about how well the heart pumps.

Nuclear scans can be used. Sometimes a positive emission tomography (**PET scan**) or a **thallium scan** is needed.

* Computerized tomography

treatment overview

These tests will help your doctor or nurse treat what's going on in your heart. Each heartbeat involves a squeeze (pumping) and time for relaxing (filling). Although pumping problems are more common*, heart failure often includes some of both of these:

> **weak pumping** *(reduced ejection fraction)*
> The ejection fraction (EF) is an estimate of the heart's pumping strength. Normal strength is 50% or higher. Less than 50% means reduced heart pumping.

> **poor filling** *(normal ejection fraction)*
> Stiff lower chambers do not relax enough for good filling and stretching. If your heart failure is mostly due to poor filling, your EF may be normal (preserved*). The heart muscle pumps well but doesn't relax enough for good filling. Filling problems are common with heart failure due to high blood pressure but can also occur with other heart problems.

When your body doesn't get enough oxygen-rich blood, stress hormones and nerve signals tell the body arteries to tighten. Tight arteries make it harder for your heart to pump. Stress hormones also keep salt and water from going out in your urine. This means fluid can build up in the tight blood vessels, making even more work for the heart. Extra salt and water in the body will cause thirst but drinking too much fluid will make things worse.

Medicines to relax tight arteries (and remove any extra fluid) will make it easier for your heart to fill and pump out the blood. Most heart failure patients also need to eat less salt to avoid fluid-buildup, reduce swelling and breathe easier.

* 2013 ACCF/AHA Guideline for the Management of Heart Failure. Circulation. 2013;128:1810-1852.

Medical Treatment

For most, the daily treatment of heart failure includes:

- ☐ **3 or more medicines and a weight record to watch for fluid buildup**

- ☐ **eating less salt and limiting fluids**

- ☐ **balancing low-level exercise and rest**

- ☐ **reducing demands on your heart when you can**

Some patients also get a daily benefit from an implanted pacemaker or ICD (see pages 18-19).

take medicines and keep a daily weight record

These four types of drugs are common in treating heart failure:

1. **ACE inhibitors and ARB's** relax your blood vessels and make your heart's workload easier over time.

2. **Beta-** or a **beta-and alpha-blocker** offer many long-term benefits to make your heart's workload easier.

3. **Diuretics** cause you to pass more urine. This helps reduce the amount of blood your heart has to pump. Some diuretics also block aldosterone (a stress hormone) and save potassium.

4. **Digoxin** may help control heart failure due to poor pumping.

Other drugs may be needed to prevent clots. This includes aspirin, an anti-platelet drug or a "blood thinner." Drugs to control heart rhythm (beta-blocker and/or anti-arrhythmic) may also be needed.

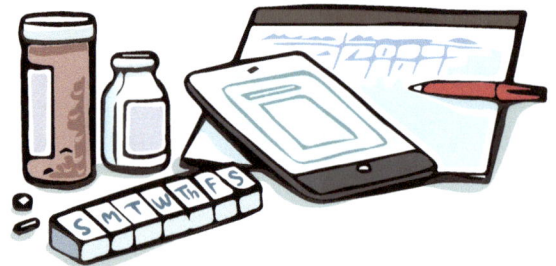

ACE inhibitors (or ARBs)

Angiotensin-converting enzyme (ACE) inhibitors are used to treat heart failure. These drugs limit the amount of angiotensin, a substance your body makes to tighten the arteries. They offer long-term benefits that help improve symptoms, keep heart failure from getting worse and prolong life.

When you begin taking an ACE inhibitor, you may feel weak, dizzy or have a cough that seems to hang on. Tell your doctor or nurse about any of these so a dosage or drug change can be made.

Non-steroidal anti-inflammatory drugs (NSAIDs) interfere with the benefits of ACE inhibitors and can worsen heart failure by causing fluid retention. Talk with your doctor or nurse before you take any NSAIDs, even over-the-counter ones like ibuprofen, Advil®, Motrin®, Aleve® and other arthritis medicines.

Angiotensin II receptor blockers (ARBs) or vasodilators are used to relax blood vessels when someone cannot take an ACE inhibitor. Both help keep heart failure from getting worse. If someone can't take an ACE inhibitor or an ARB, vasodilators may be helpful.

Some ARBs are:

> losartan (Cozaar®)

> sacubitril/valsartan (Entresto®) or valsartan (Diovan®)

> candesartan (Atacand®)

Some vasodilators are:

> nitroglycerin (Nitro-Dur®)

> hydralazine* (Apresoline®)

> isosorbide* (Isordil®)

*BiDil® is a combination of these 2 drugs, first proven helpful in African-Americans with a weak heart. BiDil® can also be helpful when someone has heart failure and cannot take an ACE inhibitor or ARB.

Ace inhibitors

Vasotec®
(enalapril)

Capoten®
(captopril)

Prinivil®
or
Zestril®
(lisinopril)

Accupril®
(quinapril)

Altace®
(ramipril)

Monopril®
(fosinopril)

You should NOT stop taking your ACE inhibitor, ARB or vasodilator drugs without your doctor or nurse's advice, no matter how good you feel.

beta- and alpha-blockers

Beta- and alpha-blocker drugs block the effect of certain nerve signals and hormones (adrenaline and norepinephrine). When these are blocked, body arteries relax and your heartbeat slows down. As the heart pumps more blood to your kidneys, sodium and extra fluid are passed in the urine. Heart failure symptoms are likely to improve after 2 to 3 months.

When you first begin to use a beta-blocker, side effects such as holding fluid, feeling more tired, a slower heartbeat or dizziness may occur. These side effects often stop and do not prevent long-term use of a beta-blocker.

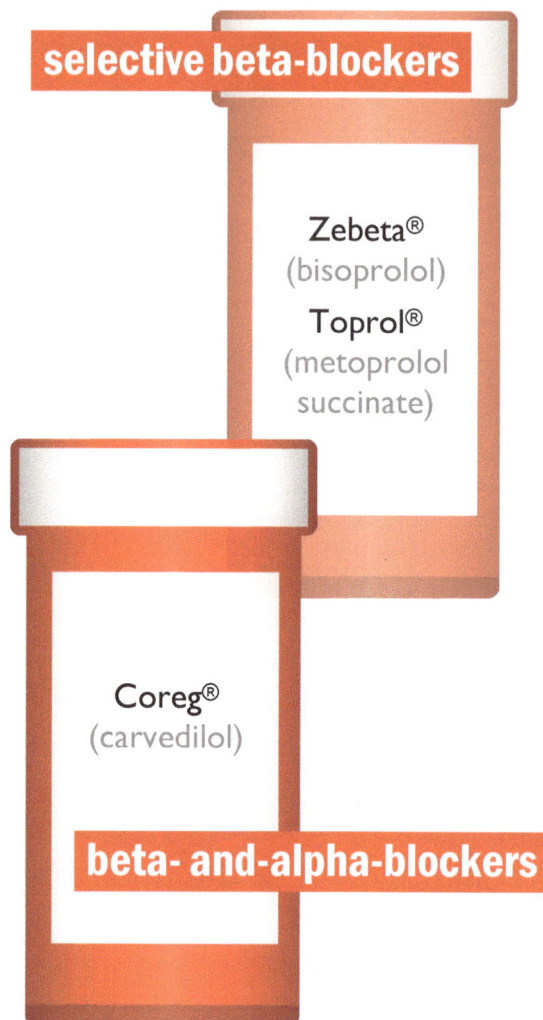

selective beta-blockers

Zebeta®
(bisoprolol)

Toprol®
(metoprolol succinate)

Coreg®
(carvedilol)

beta- and-alpha-blockers

Taking an **ACE inhibitor** or **beta-blocker** improves heart failure over time (i.e., months and years).

Studies show that people with a weak heart muscle (ejection fraction <40%) will live longer if they take an ACE inhibitor as well as a beta-blocker.

Low doses are often used at first with slow increases (every 2 to 4 weeks) to get the most benefit with the least side effects.

diuretics (and potassium supplements)

Diuretics (water pills) help the kidneys make more urine and get rid of excess fluid. Diuretics can also decrease fluid in the lungs and help you breathe more easily. But at night, you may need to go to the bathroom more. When you lie down, more blood goes to your kidneys, which causes them to make more urine.

Holding fluid is very common when the heart is not pumping well. Taking diuretics daily and limiting salt help prevent this fluid build-up.

Many people with heart failure are told to weigh daily and watch for fluid build-up (3-4 lb weight gain in 1-2 days or 2 lbs overnight). If you have fluid build-up, take action. Call your doctor or nurse right away for advice to reduce your heart's workload.

If you have fluid build-up often, you may be told to take an extra diuretic tablet. This weight chart shows one heart failure patient's success following his doctor's advice to take an extra Lasix® for rapid weight gain:

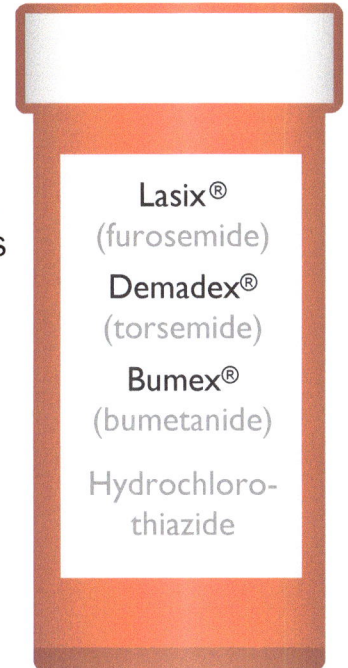

diuretics

Lasix®
(furosemide)

Demadex®
(torsemide)

Bumex®
(bumetanide)

Hydrochloro-
thiazide

example:

Date	Weight	Diuretic Taken
11/6	152 lbs	20mg Lasix® (furosemide) tablet
11/7	156 lbs	40mg Lasix® (furosemide) tablet
11/8	151 lbs	20mg Lasix® (furosemide) tablet

Always follow your doctor or nurse's advice about diuretics. Taking too much diuretic on your own can cause serious and even life-threatening problems. If you are urinating a lot, but still holding fluid—eat less salt and stop eating out.

potassium supplements

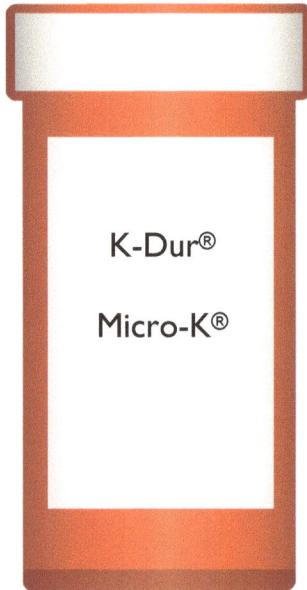

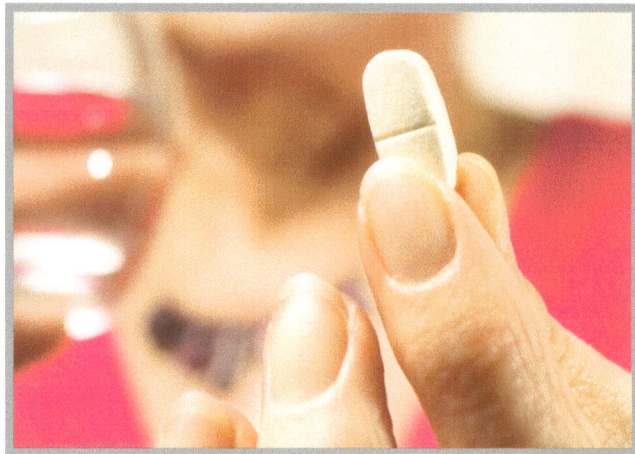

K-Dur®

Micro-K®

potassium sparing diuretics

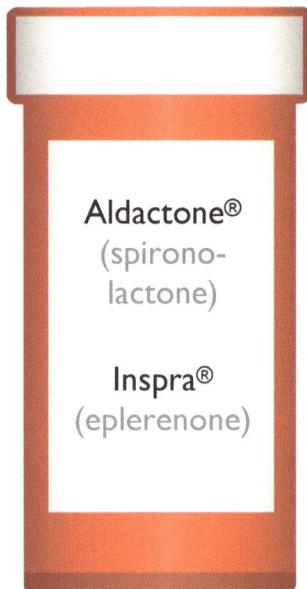

Aldactone®
(spirono-
lactone)

Inspra®
(eplerenone)

Your body needs potassium. Heart rhythm depends on a normal blood potassium (K+). Many diuretics cause a loss of potassium in the urine. Often, food alone can't replace the amount of potassium removed by the diuretic. A blood test is used to see if potassium supplements are needed. Most people who need supplements take them with their meals.

Some diuretics also block a stress hormone called aldosterone. Blocking this hormone can help keep heart failure from getting worse. Spironolactone (Aldactone®) and eplerenone (Inspra®) are examples of aldosterone-blocker diuretics*. Unlike most other diuretics, aldosterone-blocker diuretics are 'potassium-sparing'. Taking a potassium-sparing diuretic may mean taking fewer potassium supplements (or none in some cases). Blood tests to monitor potassium are needed, especially after the first 7 days of taking a potassium-sparing diuretic.

Blood tests also show if kidney function changes over time. This can happen with heart failure, causing you to need less potassium. Some people with heart failure **do not** need any extra potassium. They are told to avoid salt substitutes and sodium-free bouillon since both are high in potassium.

 * Males who get breast tenderness while taking an aldosterone-blocker diuretic should tell their doctor or nurse. Often a different potassium-sparing diuretic can be used without this side effect.

High potassium foods

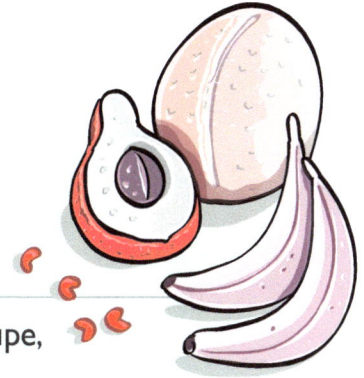

dried fruits	raisins, prunes, apricots, dates
fresh fruits	bananas, watermelon, cantaloupe, oranges, kiwi, nectarines
fresh vegetables	avocados, potatoes, broccoli, greens, spinach, tomatoes, mushroom
dried vegetables	beans, peas
fresh juices	orange
canned juices	prune, apricot NOTE: Avoid canned juices, like tomato and V-8®, that contain salt. Read all labels for salt, sodium or sodium compounds (or NaCl, as salt is often written).
salt substitutes or sodium-free bouillon (Often high in potassium)	NOTE: Check with your doctor or nurse before using salt substitutes or sodium-free bouillon. Most have a lot of potassium and in some people, too much potassium can be dangerous.

Remember—diuretics send extra body fluid out in the urine, often washing out potassium at the same time. Regular blood tests for potassium are needed to see if you need to eat more high-potassium foods or if you should avoid those foods. Do what your doctor or nurse tells you to keep your potassium within healthy levels.

digoxin

Digoxin (Lanoxin®) may help control heart failure in people with reduced heart pumping. Studies show it may also prevent hospital re-admissions. If you still have symptoms after taking an ACE inhibitor (or ARB), a beta-blocker, and a diuretic(s), digoxin may be used. Digoxin can also be used for irregular heart rhythms such as atrial fibrillation.

Sometimes digoxin builds up in the body. This can cause one or more of these:

- loss of appetite, distaste for food or a bad taste in the mouth

- nausea or vomiting

- blue or yellow vision

- skipped heartbeats, palpitations or rapid beating

If any of these occur, tell your doctor or nurse right away. Too much digoxin can cause other heart rhythm problems. Be sure to take it only as your doctor or nurse orders.

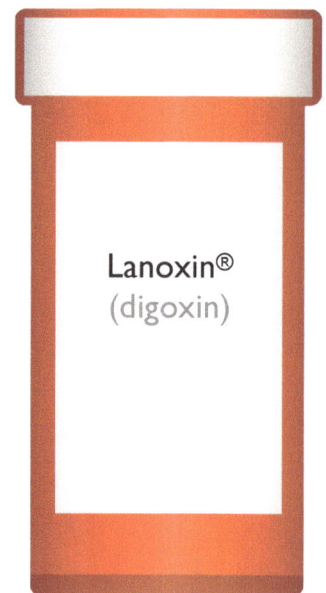

Lanoxin®
(digoxin)

other drugs

Some heart failure patients also need medicine to reduce the risk of blood clots, to control rapid heart rates (often a beta-blocker) or to prevent an abnormal heart rhythm (anti-arrhythmic).

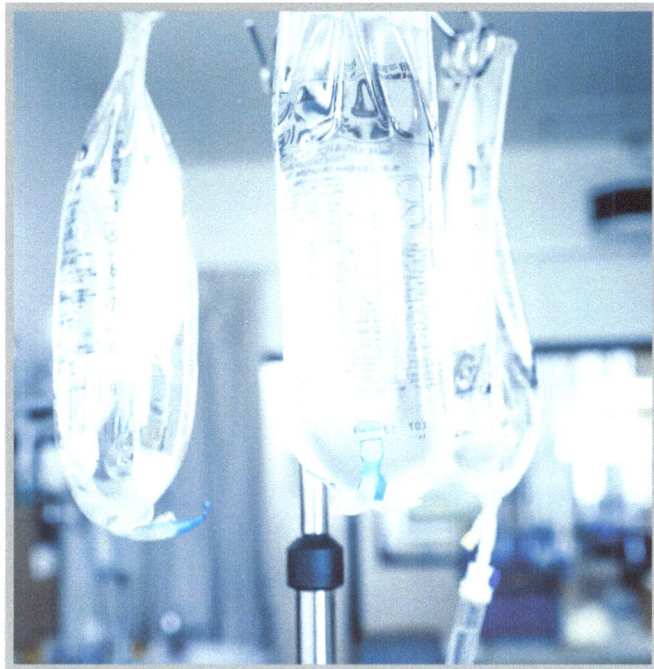

in-hospital drugs or procedures

IV medicine

Sometimes intravenous (IV) drugs are used for short-term relief of severe or sudden onset heart failure. IV diuretics can help the kidneys quickly remove extra fluid. Drugs to prevent blood clots (example: Heparin) can be given by IV in the hospital. Blood tests are used to monitor the dose.

IV drugs like dobutamine and milrinone can make your heart beat stronger. IV nesiritide (Natrecor®) can make it easier for your heart to pump by relaxing your arteries and causing your kidneys to remove extra fluid.

These drugs are given through a small tube in your vein. Often a pump controls how much medicine you get. Blood pressure checks are often needed when you get these IV drugs.

Ultrafiltration

Sometimes a procedure called ultrafiltration is used to remove the extra fluid when diuretics and other treatments aren't working. Ultrafiltration involves passing the blood through a special filter so excess salt and fluid can be removed.

Surgery for heart failure

coronary artery bypass graft (CABG)

Sometimes heart bypass surgery can help blood flow to the heart when artery blockage is about to cause heart damage. Although more blood flow doesn't help areas of old damage (scar), bypass surgery can help limit new damage.

cardiac electrical devices

Your doctor will let you know if your heart failure can be improved with a cardiac electrical device. This could include:

> a biventricular pacemaker to correct an electrical delay

and/or

> an internal defibrillator (ICD) to help stop a life-threatening heart rhythm

Often heart failure patients need a device that works as both a pacemaker and a defibrillator.

Pacemaker (biventricular or CRT*)

Some heart failure patients have an electrical delay in their heart muscle contractions. This delay may mean the heart chambers do not beat when they should. If you have this delay, a biventricular pacemaker can correct it, so the chambers can beat in normal sequence. This may improve your heart failure symptoms and give you more energy.

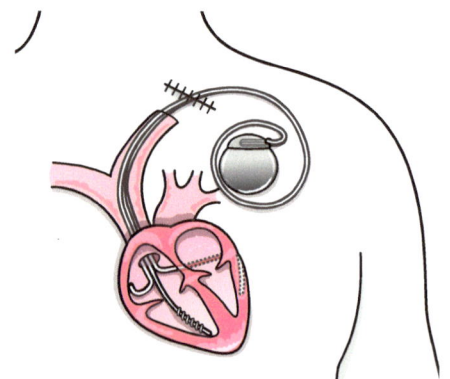

* Biventricular pacing is also known as cardiac resynchronization therapy (CRT).

Internal Cardioverter Defibrillator (ICD)

An ICD is used to stop life-threatening heart rhythms. The device can tell when these rhythms occur. Within seconds, it can give a shock and try to stop the rhythm.

Recent studies have shown that an ICD can help someone with heart failure who is at risk for a life-threatening heart rhythm. Most ICDs can also pace your heart to help keep a normal rhythm.

A few precautions are advised if you have a cardiac device. **Large electromagnetic fields must be avoided, especially if you have an ICD.** More information is available on the device maker's website and the Pritchett & Hull booklet, **You Have a Pacemaker and/or ICD.**

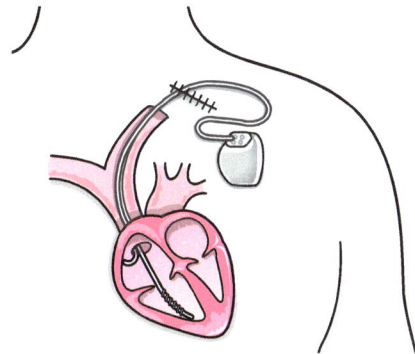

All cardiac devices require regular follow-up. Often wireless technology and/or phone lines allow you to send device readings from home to a secure internet server for your doctor or clinic to review. Your doctor is notified right away of important changes. Sometimes weight and blood pressure readings are also sent through the home monitoring system. Your healthcare provider can see changes in your readings and may be able to adjust your medication before you have major symptoms or need a hospital stay.

VAD (ventricular assist device)

A ventricular assist device (VAD) refers to a small pump placed in the chest to boost blood flow from a lower heart chamber to a large body artery. Newer VADS are smaller* and often allow living at home with family support. VAD patients often have more energy, fewer medications and an improved quality of life. A VAD can be implanted for long-term use (destination therapy).

All of today's VAD pumps have a **drive-line tubing** that comes through the skin and connects to a small outside VAD computer. Cables from the VAD computer lead to either **battery or AC power.** During the day the batteries and VAD computer are placed in a bag or the pockets of a VAD vest worn over clothing. At night, the patient (and family) disconnect the battery cables and plug them into the AC-powered VAD cable.

The VAD patient or family member do the regular sterile dressing changes needed to prevent infection where the drive-line tubing comes through the skin. Although showers are OK, **swimming and tub bathing are not allowed** with a VAD. Prior to a shower, place a company-specific product over the dressing like the ShowerGuard® by Centurion or plastic wrap like Glad Press'N'Seal®. The batteries and VAD computer go in a 'shower kit' provided by the device company. Many activities are fine for someone with a VAD as long as there is **no tension on the drive-line tubing. Contact sports are NOT ok.**

Continuous-Flow VAD

pump (inside body)

batteries

VAD tubing (drive-line)

VAD computer

* HeartMate II® VAD made by Thoratec® is only 3 inches long and weighs 10 ounces.

heart transplant

Heart transplants replace a failing heart that can no longer meet the body's needs. The stress of heart transplant surgery and the side effects of anti-rejection medicine put a serious strain on certain body functions. So the surgery is limited to those with severe heart failure who qualify for transplant and otherwise have healthy body organs. Costly medicines and life-long medical follow-up are needed to prevent the body from rejecting the new heart. The need for heart transplants far exceeds the number of donor organs.

In some cases, a ventricular assist device (VAD) can be used as temporary support for someone who isn't doing well enough to wait for a heart donor. In this case, the VAD is used as a "bridge" to transplantation. Research continues to find ways to:

> help a damaged heart heal itself (gene therapy and/or stem cell injections),

> wrap or reshape heart chambers, and

> perfect a mechanical device that will fully support heart function.

Controlling the symptoms and stress of a serious illness can be difficult. If your doctor suggests **palliative care**, you can get extra help with:

- symptom management (anxiety; constipation, diarrhea or nausea; difficulty breathing, sleeping or eating)

- making difficult health decisions and finding community resources that can help you at home

A palliative care team often includes a doctor, nurse, social worker and/or chaplain. All can consult with your primary heart failure doctor as needed.

Your role in heart failure control

step 1: take your medicines exactly as prescribed

☐ Have a written schedule and a pill box or another way to remember your medicine.

☐ Report any side effects to your doctor or nurse (dizziness, loss of appetite, nausea or changes in mental or sexual function). **Do not stop taking any of your medicine on your own.**

☐ Take your diuretic in the morning to limit bathroom trips at night. If you take a diuretic twice a day, ask your doctor or nurse about spacing the second dose in the late afternoon.

☐ If you miss a dose, don't take extra to make up for it. But if you forget your diuretic in the morning, take it later in the day rather than waiting until the next morning.

☐ Once you feel better, don't stop any of your medicines! Many of them work best together for a good long-term effect on the heart and blood vessels.

☐ Talk to your doctor or nurse before taking any herbs or other supplements. Some may interfere with your medicines, especially the blood thinner Coumadin® (warfarin) or, in a few cases, Pradaxa® (dabigatran).

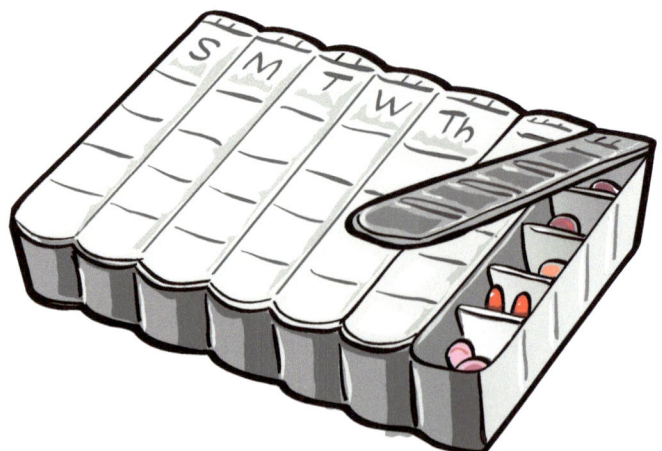

⊙ Check the zero point
on your scale each
time you use it.

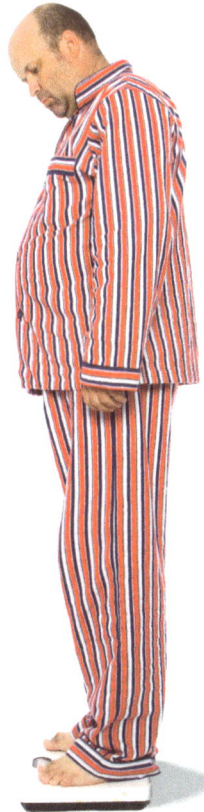

step 2: weigh daily and watch for rapid fluid buildup

☐ When home, always use the same scale. Keep it adjusted to zero. Use it on a hard surface (not carpet) each time. When you travel, make sure you have a good scale to weigh on.

☐ Weigh yourself each morning. Do this after urinating, but before eating or getting dressed. **Keep a written record to take to your doctor or nurse.**

☐ Report any rapid weight gain to your doctor or nurse (example: 3–4 pounds in 1–2 days of normal eating or 2 pounds overnight).

☐ If you have been eating the same amount of food, a quick weight gain is often a sign that fluid is building up and causing more work for your heart.

☐ Follow your doctor's or nurse's advice about a sudden weight gain. You may need more diuretic and/or potassium supplements. **Do not take more without your doctor's or nurse's advice.**

step 3: eat less salt and limit fluid intake

Since foods high in sodium (salt) make the body hold fluid, eat less of them. The average American takes in around 3,300 mg sodium per day.* It's easy to see why, since one teaspoon of table salt has about 2,300 mg of sodium. Most of our sodium intake doesn't come from the salt shaker. We get large amounts in fast or processed food, large restaurant meals and high-sodium spices. Read food labels and learn about packaged foods and the spices high in sodium. Some people with heart failure do well on 2,400–3,000 mg of sodium a day, but most must limit sodium to less than 2,000 mg/day.

Many people with heart failure have trouble with their body holding fluid. Being very thirsty is also common because diuretics take away the extra fluid. **Even if you are thirsty, DO NOT** replace all the fluid that diuretics have helped your body get rid of. Use small amounts of hard sugar-free candy to help with a dry mouth.

Your doctor or nurse may tell you to have no more than 2 quarts (64 ounces) of fluid per day (or less in some cases). This includes **all beverages**, high-moisture foods/fruits, Jell-O®, ice cream and ice cubes (see page 28).

Following your doctor or nurse's advice about sodium and fluids can help you control heart failure and take less diuretic.

* *What We Eat in America,*
 U.S. Department of Agriculture.

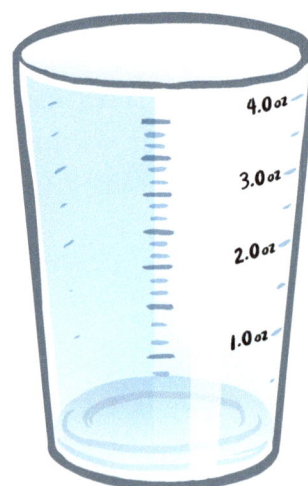

4.0 oz

3.0 oz

2.0 oz

1.0 oz

Hints to lower sodium in your diet

> **Do not cook with salt** or add salt to foods at the table.

> **Eat fresh vegetables or unsalted canned or frozen vegetables.** These have less sodium than most processed foods. For example:*

Instead Of:	Eat
1 cup of regular canned peas: 400 mg of sodium	1 cup of fresh, cooked peas; 2 mg of sodium

*Sodium content of foods from USDA Handbook #456.

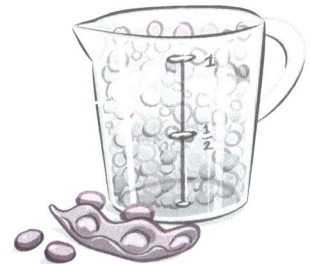

> **Season with fresh or dried herbs, vegetables or no-salt seasonings.**

> **Bake, broil, boil, steam, roast** or **poach** foods without salt. Eat out rarely, but when you do, order foods cooked without breading, butter or sauces. Ask that no salt be added. Don't eat soups (usually high in sodium). Go easy on the salad dressing as most are high in salt. Don't eat at restaurants that cause you to have a sudden weight gain the next day.

> **Make your own** sauces, salad dressings, vegetable dishes and desserts when you can. Some patients make their own bread to further lower sodium intake.

> **When buying canned fish, low-sodium tuna or salmon is best.** You can use water-packed tuna or salmon if you break it up and soak it for 3 minutes in cold water. Rinse, drain and squeeze out the water.

Keep track of your sodium intake each day. It may surprise you how fast it adds up. Follow your doctor or nurse's advice to limit sodium and buy mostly low-sodium foods (see next page).

Low-sodium foods—what you CAN eat (✔)

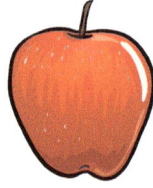

fruits and vegetables

✔ fresh or frozen (check for sodium)

✔ canned (unsalted)

drinks

✔ fruit juices, fresh or frozen

✔ canned low-sodium or no salt added tomato and vegetable juice

✔ instant breakfast (all flavors but eggnog)— limit to 1 cup/day

✔ frozen concentrate or fresh lemonade

dairy choices

✔ up to 3 cups of your daily fluid allotment in milk (1%, skim or homemade buttermilk using baking buttermilk powder)

✔ no-salt added cottage cheese

✔ ricotta—part skim, up to ½ cup a day

✔ up to 1 oz a day— hard cheeses like unprocessed Swiss, part-skim Mozzarella, Neufchâtel or string

✔ soft margarine or mayonnaise (up to 2 Tbsp a day)

✔ non-fat and low-fat sour cream

meats, poultry, fish & meat substitutes

✔ fish, fresh or frozen (not breaded); canned tuna and salmon (unsalted or rinsed)

✔ chicken or turkey (not processed in salt solution)

✔ lean cuts of beef, veal, pork, lamb

✔ dried beans, peas, lentils (not canned unless low-sodium)

✔ nuts or seeds (unsalted, dry roasted)

✔ unsalted peanut butter, up to 2 Tbsp a day

✔ tofu (soybean curd)

    * Using homemade breads (no self-rising flour) can reduce sodium intake further.

breads, cereals, grains

✔ loaf bread and yeast rolls (3 slices/ day)*

✔ melba toast, matzo crackers

✔ pita bread, taco shells or corn tortillas

✔ cooked cereals (avoid instant): corn grits, farina (regular), oatmeal, oat bran, cream of rice or wheat

✔ puffed rice or wheat, shredded wheat (or any cereal with 100–150 mg sodium—limit to 1 cup/day)

✔ wheat germ

✔ popcorn (no salt or fat added)

✔ rice (enriched white or brown) or pasta

cooking ingredients, seasonings

✔ corn starch, tapioca

✔ corn meal or flour (not self-rising)

✔ fresh or dried herbs, salt-free herb seasonings

✔ lemons, limes, onions, celery

✔ fresh garlic, ginger or vinegar

✔ Louisiana-type hot sauce (1 tsp/day)

✔ low-sodium baking powder, yeast, onion or garlic powder

✔ tomato paste, unsalted tomatoes, unsalted tomato sauce

✔ water chestnuts

✔ carob powder, cocoa powder

✔ low sodium salad dressings

sweets

✔ flavored gelatins

✔ frozen juice bars, fruit ice, sorbet, sherbet

✔ sugar, honey, molasses, syrup

✔ jelly, jams, preserves, apple butter

✔ graham and animal crackers, fig bars, ginger snaps

Read food labels

Until you learn how to eat a low-sodium diet, add up the sodium content in all the foods and beverages you take in per day. Be sure it is less than your doctor or nurse has advised. Tips to help you:

> Buy products labeled low-sodium, sodium-free, or very low sodium. At present, a "low-sodium" food label means 140 mg of sodium* or less per serving size.

> Pay attention to the serving size as you figure the amount you plan to eat. Sometimes the food label shows the sodium mg for only a tiny amount of food rather than a common serving size. Labels like "healthy", "reduced sodium", "unsalted", "no salt added" or "without added salt" can also be misleading.

> Always count the sodium content for the amount of food you plan to eat! Sometimes the food label shows the sodium mg for only a tiny amount of food rather than a common serving size. Use caution even if you see food labels like "healthy", "reduced sodium", "unsalted", "no salt added" or "without added salt".

> Studies show that 75-80% of our daily sodium intake comes from processed and restaurant foods. When possible, avoid eating out. Ask family or friends not to add salt to your food. Almost all fast food is high in salt. Don't buy convenience foods like prepared or skillet dinners, deli food, cold cuts, hot dogs, most frozen entrees or canned soups.

* www.fda.gov

Nutrition Facts

Serving Size 1 hotdog link (57 grams)
Servings Per Container 8

Amount Per Serving

Calories 170	Calories from Fat 140

% Daily Value*

Total Fat 16g	25%
Saturated Fat 5g	25%
Trans Fat 0g	
Cholesterol 45 mg	15%
Sodium 480 mg	20%
Total Carbohydrate <1g	0%
Protein 6g	

Vitamin C	20%	•	Iron	6%
Calcium	6%			

* Percent Daily Values are based on a 2,000 calorie diet. Your daily values may be higher or lower depending on your calorie needs:

	Calories	2,000	2,500
Total Fat	Less than	65g	80g
Sat Fat	Less than	20g	25g
Cholesterol	Less than	300mg	300mg
Sodium	Less than	2,400mg	2,400mg
Total Carbohydrate		300g	375g
Dietary Fiber		25g	30g

1g Fat = 9 calories
1g Carbohydrates = 4 calories
1 g Protein = 4 calories

High-sodium foods—what NOT to eat (✘)

vegetables
✘ salted canned vegetables
✘ sauerkraut

breads, cereals, grains, starches
✘ self-rising flour and corn meal
✘ prepared mixes (Ex: waffle, pancake, muffin, cornbread and all frozen waffles)
✘ instant cooked cereals

dairy products
✘ buttermilk (store-bought)
✘ canned milk (unless diluted and used as regular milk)
✘ egg substitute (limit to ½ cup/day)
✘ eggnog (store-bought)
✘ salted butter and margarine with transfat
✘ certain cheese (American and other processed cheese, blue cheese, Parmesan, feta and regular cottage cheese) with more than 200 mg/serving

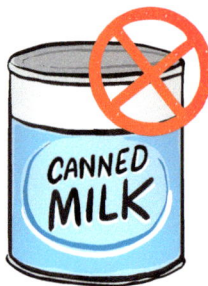

soups
✘ bouillon (all kinds)
✘ dry soup mixes
✘ canned broth and soups* (with more than 350 mg sodium/serving)

drinks
✘ athletic drinks (such as Gatorade®)
✘ canned tomato or vegetable juice (unless unsalted)

sweets
✘ prepared mixes or store-bought pies, puddings, cakes, muffins, etc.

meats and meat substitutes
✘ canned meats and fish (sardines, unrinsed tuna and salmon)
✘ cured meats (Ex: dried beef, bacon, corned beef) and any meat product processed with salt (ham, some chicken and pork)
✘ all types sausage and hot dogs (Ex: beef, pork, chicken, turkey, Polish sausage, hot dogs, knockwurst)
✘ rotisserie chicken
✘ sandwich meats (bologna, salami, olive loaf, etc.)
✘ regular peanut butter
✘ salted nuts

cooking ingredients, seasonings, condiments, snacks
✘ fermented miso and cooking wine
✘ pre-seasoned mixes for tacos, spaghetti, chili, etc.
✘ coating mixes
✘ preseasoned convenience foods
✘ soy, teriyaki or Asian fish sauce
✘ baking soda, baking powder (use low-sodium type)
✘ olives, pickles (dill, sour, sweet gherkins)
✘ pretzels, chips, skins, etc.
✘ light salt, seasoning salt, sea salt, meat tenderizer, garlic salt, monosodium glutamate (MSG), kosher salt, celery salt, onion salt, lemon pepper

Note: Check the label. Use less than 2 Tbsp a day of tomato sauce (unless unsalted), catsup, chili sauce, BBQ sauce, mustard or salad dressings.

* Even reduced sodium canned soups can be quite high in salt. Check the label.

Follow your doctor or nurse's advice about limiting salt and fluid intake. Some people with heart failure do well on 2,400 mg of sodium a day, but most must limit daily sodium to less than 2,000 mg to avoid fluid buildup.

Your doctor or nurse may ask you to limit liquids to 2 quarts (64oz) a day. The liquid content of high moisture food has to be counted as well as all beverages, liquid with medicine and ice cubes. Ice cubes usually melt to half their size: 4oz ice=2 oz fluid. Refer to the moisture content of the food examples in this list. Ask your doctor or nurse if you need more help keeping your total fluid intake to 2 quarts.

Food examples of liquid content/serving size:

FOOD	LIQUID	FOOD	LIQUID
½ cup ice cream or sherbet	2 oz	15 grapes	1 oz
3 oz popsicle	2 oz	½ cup cherries or medium-size lemon	2 oz
½ cup fruited Jell-O®	3 oz	9 inch banana or medium-size peach	2.5 oz
½ cup pudding or custard	3.5 oz		
1 cup low-sodium broth-based soup	7 oz	½ cup applesauce, canned peaches, pears or pineapple	3 oz
1 cup yogurt, low-sodium cream soup or can of nutritional supplement	6 oz	½ cup fruit cocktail	3.5 oz
medium-size pear	4.5 oz	Medium-size apple, nectarine, orange, or 1 cup strawberries	4 oz
1 cup watermelon	5 oz		

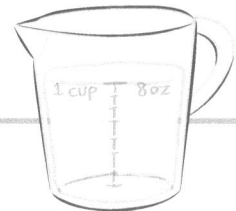

Even if you are <u>NOT</u> told to restrict fluids, avoid large amounts of high moisture foods.

step 4: find the right balance in exercise and rest for you

> **Rest throughout your day.** Put your feet up for a few minutes throughout your day. Consider a nap after lunch.

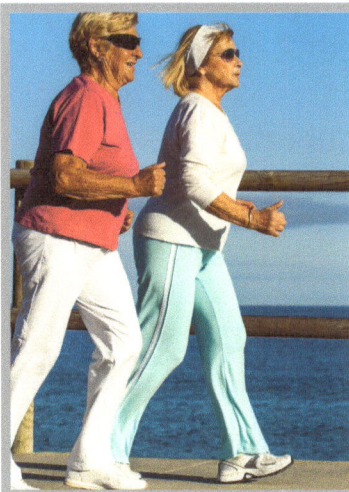

> **After talking with your doctor or nurse, begin walking or another exercise that you enjoy.** Exercise often lessens bad feelings and gives you more energy and quality of life. Walking on a treadmill, bicycling and swimming allow you to use the large muscle groups. Find an exercise that doesn't make you too tired and one that doesn't keep you from talking while doing it. Don't lift really heavy objects. Strength training is good but ask your doctor or nurse before you start.

step 5: make less work for your heart when you can

☐ **Reduce high blood pressure.** Ask your doctor or nurse for your blood pressure goal and how to reach it.

☐ **Get rid of any excess body fat.** Find healthy ways to lose fat (if needed) and keep a normal body weight. Bodies that are too large put more demand on the heart.

☐ **Control diabetes by keeping your blood sugar (A1C level) in the range your doctor or nurse suggests.** Ask if any of your diabetic drugs are likely to lead to fluid buildup.

☐ **Stop smoking!!!** All tobacco products tighten body arteries and make more work for your heart. Talk to your doctor or nurse if you need help quitting.

☐ **If you snore or are sleepy throughout the day, tell your doctor or nurse.** A sleep study may be needed to see if you have pauses in breathing (sleep apnea).

☐ **Ask your doctor or nurse if you can have alcohol.** Since alcohol weakens the heart, heart failure may improve if you stop drinking.

☐ **Reduce emotional stress.** You may feel depressed, angry or anxious because you have heart failure. Talking about your feelings, exercise, meditation and/or medicine may help.

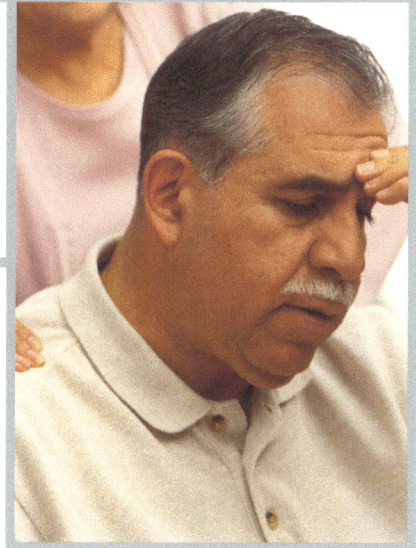

☐ **Avoid temperature extremes.** The body works harder to keep a normal temperature when you're too hot or cold.

☐ **Reduce high cholesterol levels** to prevent fatty buildup and damage to your arteries. Many need to take a "statin", omega-3 fatty acid, or another anti-cholesterol drug.

☐ **Stay away from people who have colds or flu.** Ask your doctor or nurse to keep you up-to-date with flu and pneumonia vaccines.

☐ **Avoid blood clots.** Regular walking and not wearing garters or hose with tight tops help improve blood flow in the legs. Your doctor or nurse may also tell you to wear special stockings. An irregular heart rhythm (atrial fibrillation) can occur along with heart failure, adding to the risk of a blood clot. You may be asked to take 1 or more drugs to prevent blood clots:

> aspirin

> an anti-platelet drug like Plavix® (clopidogrel), Effient® (prasugrel) or Brilinta® (ticagrelor)

   OR

> a 'blood thinner' like Coumadin® (warfarin), Eliquis® (apixaban), Pradaxa® (dabigatran), Xarelto® (rivaroxaban) or Savaysa® (edoxaban).

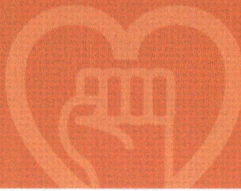

In Summary

You have the most important role in managing your heart failure. Having a partner who supports you and seeing a cardiologist or nurse practitioner who specializes in heart failure can also be helpful. Write down what you are told for home care in the space below.

Take your heart failure medicines exactly as prescribed.

Keep a medicine chart. Note directions on your prescription bottles. Some may ask you to increase the dosage gradually.

Name	Dose	How Often

Weigh daily.

Using the same scale and amount of clothing, weigh first thing each morning after urinating. Keep a written record. Follow your doctor or nurse's instructions if you have rapid weight gain.

_____ 2-3 lbs overnight **or** _____ 3-4 lbs in 1-2 days **or** _____ lbs in _____ days

Limit fluid: _____ 2 quarts/day (64 oz) **or** as your MD directs: _____ quarts/day

Limit salt intake: _____ 1500 mg/day _____ 2000 mg/day _____ 2300 mg/day

Other diet advice: _____

Find the right balance in exercise and rest.

Ask your doctor or nurse about these exercises:

☐ walking ☐ swimming ☐ bicycling ☐ treadmill ☐ elliptical

Make it easier on your heart by:

☐ **not** smoking

☐ controlling high blood pressure, diabetes or breathing problems with sleep

☐ getting rid of excess weight

Call your doctor or nurse if you have any of these new symptoms (or if they become more severe):

› Sudden weight gain (2 lbs overnight or 3-4 lbs in 1-2 days)

• Pain in belly (abdomen) or bloating

› Shortness of breath

• Chest pain/pressure

› Swelling of feet and/or hands

• Constant cough

› Bleeding or bruising easily

• Dizziness/fainting

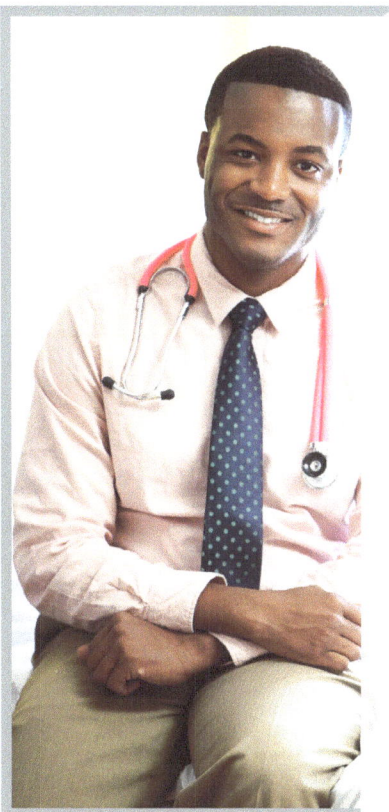

Keep appointments for blood tests and other follow-up.

› Electrolytes (sodium [Na+] and potassium [K+])

› Protime (PT) with INR (if on Coumadin® [warfarin])

› Thyroid blood level and eye, liver and lung exams (if on amiodarone to control heart rhythm)

› Other testing:_____

› Next appointment:_____

Tell your doctor about anything that bothers you during daily activity. Let them know if symptoms are keeping you from doing things you'd like to do.

Causes of heart failure

If the cause of heart failure is known, treatment can often be given for this heart problem. This offers the best long-term results. Heart failure can be temporary if the cause can be reversed. Having diabetes with or without heart disease or high blood pressure increases the risk of heart failure, especially in women.

If your healthcare provider has discussed any of these as a possible cause for your heart failure, you may want to read that page.

Cause

Note: Heart failure can also occur in adults who were born with a heart defect including some of those who had a surgical repair. See page 40 and inside back cover.

coronary heart disease

Coronary heart disease (CHD) is a buildup of cholesterol and fatty deposits in the arteries that supply the heart muscle with blood and oxygen. As these arteries become clogged, less blood reaches the heart muscle.

Heart attacks damage the heart muscle. When large areas of the heart are damaged, the remaining 'good' heart muscle has to work harder pumping out the blood. Over time the heart chambers stretch (dilate) and the heart muscle gets larger (hypertrophy). This is called cardiac remodeling and can lead to heart failure. Studies continue to find ways to slow or prevent this.

Ways to prevent CHD:

- Do not smoke

- Control blood cholesterol levels

- Control blood pressure

- Keep a healthy weight

- Exercise regularly

- Control blood sugar (for diabetes)

- Reduce stress levels

aorta

pulmonary artery

healthy muscle

blockage causes damage to heart

large damaged areas (heart attack) do not help pump

damage

remaining healthy heart muscle tries to do all the pumping

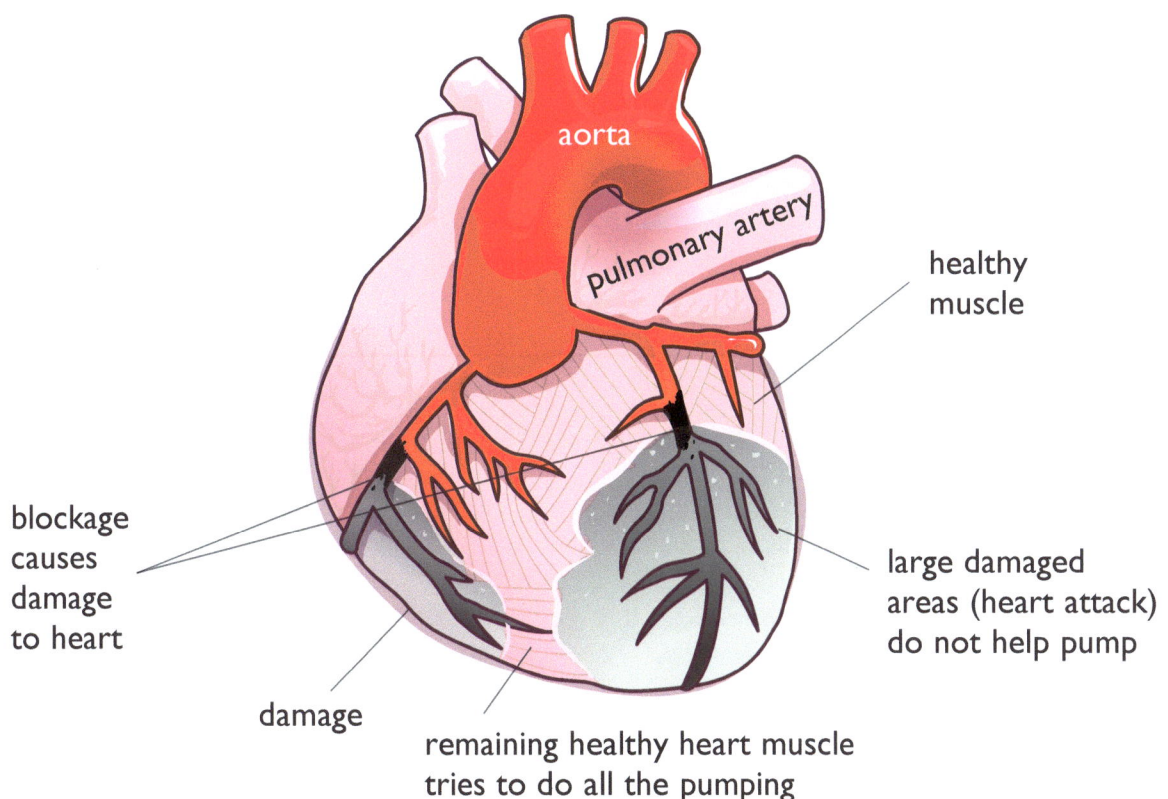

* also known as coronary artery disease or ischemic heart disease.

high blood pressure

The left lower heart (ventricle) pumps blood through the arteries carrying blood to all parts of the body. If pressure in the arteries is normal, they stretch easily and there is no extra strain on the left heart. If pressure in the arteries is high, the left heart has to pump harder to force out the blood. If blood pressure stays high for a long time, the heart muscle can weaken and heart failure can occur.

Do what your doctor or nurse says to keep your blood pressure normal. Have it checked on a regular basis. Good blood pressure control lowers the risk of new episodes of heart failure. Over 70% of Americans will develop high blood pressure in their lifetime.* The American Heart Association says people who eat less than 1,500 mg/day of sodium are not as likely to get high blood pressure. Exceptions are people who lose large amounts of sodium in sweat (athletes, workers exposed to high heat, etc). [www.heart.org]

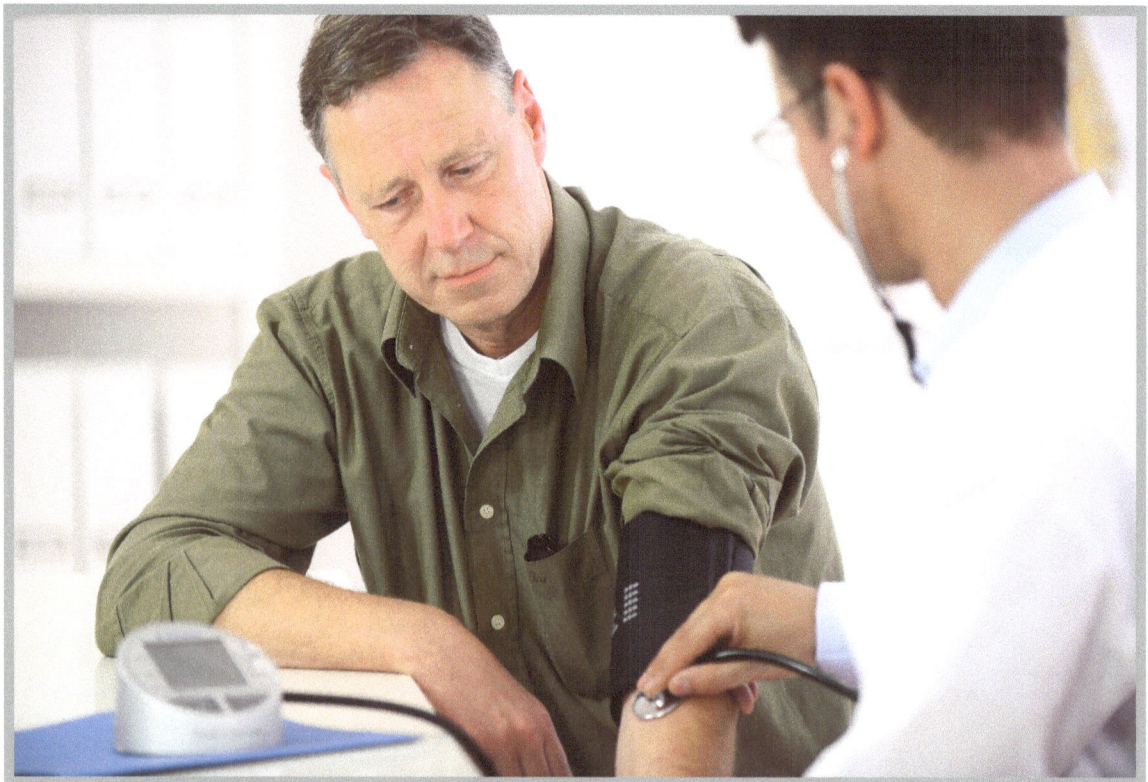

* 2013 ACCF/AHA Guidelines for the Management of Heart Failure. Circulation, 2013;128,1810-1852.)

cardiomyopathy

Cardiomyopathy is a general term for a disease of the heart muscle. You may be told that your problem is **idiopathic** (the cause is not known), or your doctor may say you have: **dilated, restrictive or hypertrophic cardiomyopathy.**

Dilated cardiomyopathy is the most common, and refers to the heart stretching or becoming larger. Viruses, the effects of alcohol or other toxic agents* or sometimes pregnancy can cause this.

Studies show that dilated cardiomyopathy tends to run in families. If the heart becomes strained, it will most often appear enlarged on a chest x-ray.

Some things can also get into the heart muscle (example: iron, amyloid [body protein] or a tumor). A stretched heart does not pump as well as it should. It is like a rubber band that has lost its snap.

Restrictive and hypertrophic cardiomyopathy often begin by making it harder for the heart to fill. A chest x-ray may not show the problem. Other tests may be needed to find out what is going on and how best to treat it.

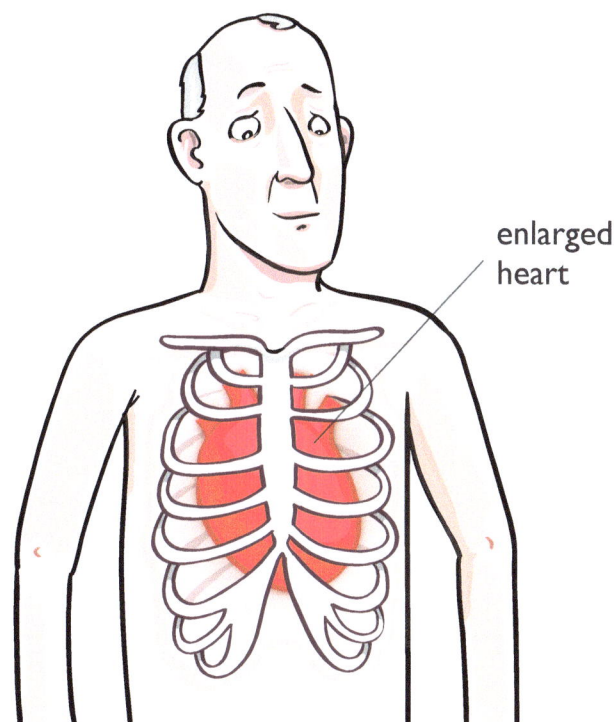

enlarged heart

* Toxic agents include illicit drugs like cocaine, methamphetamine, as well as anthracycline (Adriamycin®) or cyclophosphamide (Cytoxan) (types of chemo), ephedra (for weight loss), and Herceptin® (antibody for breast cancer).

abnormal heart valves

Abnormal heart valves are those that do not fully open or close during each heartbeat. The problem can be present at birth or due to other causes like an infection with rheumatic fever.

Normal heart valves act like doors. They open and close at the right time to move the blood forward and keep it from going backward. If a valve doesn't open or close like it should, the heart muscle has to pump harder. If the work load becomes too great, heart failure results. Sometimes surgery is needed to replace or repair a heart valve. Other times, a catheter procedure is done to help open a tight valve (TAVI® or TAVR®).

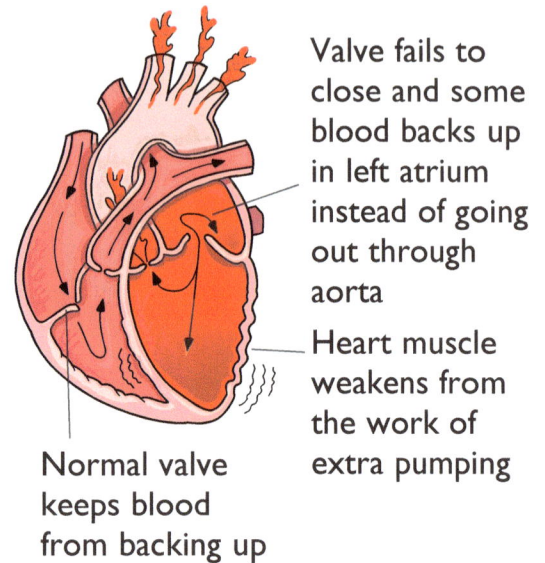

Valve fails to close and some blood backs up in left atrium instead of going out through aorta

Heart muscle weakens from the work of extra pumping

Normal valve keeps blood from backing up

severe lung disease

Severe lung disease adds to the work of the heart. If you have a chronic lung disease, treatment for it is very important. As your breathing improves, it is easier for the heart to pump blood to your lungs and body.

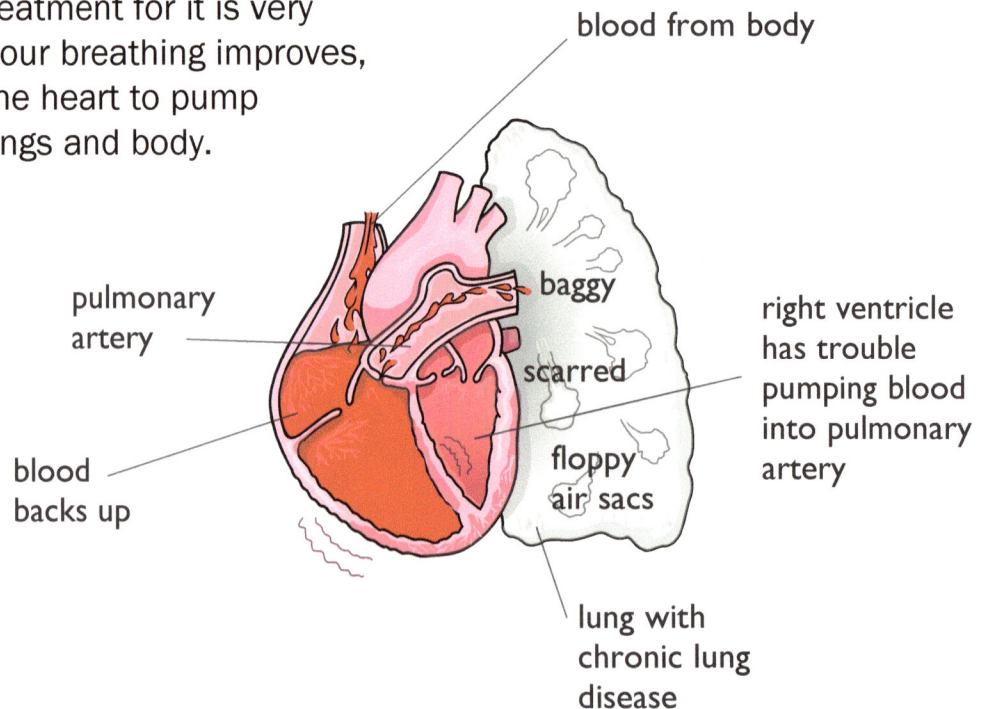

blood from body

pulmonary artery

baggy

scarred

right ventricle has trouble pumping blood into pulmonary artery

blood backs up

floppy air sacs

lung with chronic lung disease

severe anemia

Severe anemia means not having enough red blood cells to carry oxygen. The heart tries to move the small number of red blood cells at a faster rate. It can become very tired from this effort. Taking iron tablets to build more red blood cells may allow the heart to slow down and return to the normal pumping effort.

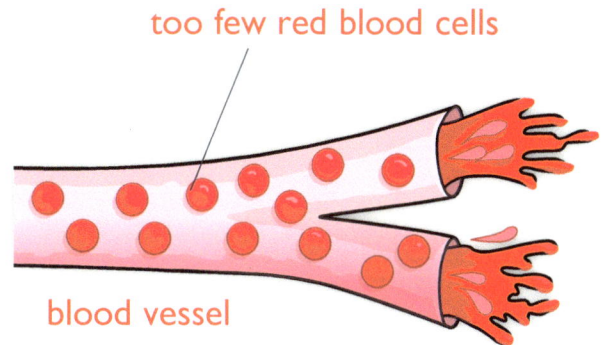

too few red blood cells

blood vessel

Anemia

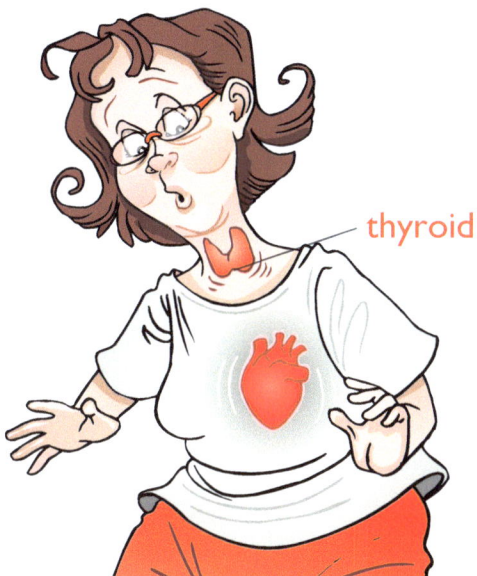

overactive thyroid

thyroid

An **overactive thyroid** gland causes the body to work at a fast pace. Over time, the heart can have trouble keeping up. Once the thyroid hormone is down to normal levels, the heart is likely to pump at a normal speed.

abnormal heart rhythm

An **abnormal heart rhythm** (arrhythmia) refers to the heart beating either too fast or too slow. In either case, the heart may not be able to pump enough blood for all of the body. Sometimes strain or heart failure may occur.

over-use of alcohol

Over-use of alcohol can weaken the heart's pumping action. If you stop drinking alcohol early enough, the heart may return to its normal strength. Doctors often suggest heart failure patients reduce or stop alcohol intake altogether.

Congenital heart disease

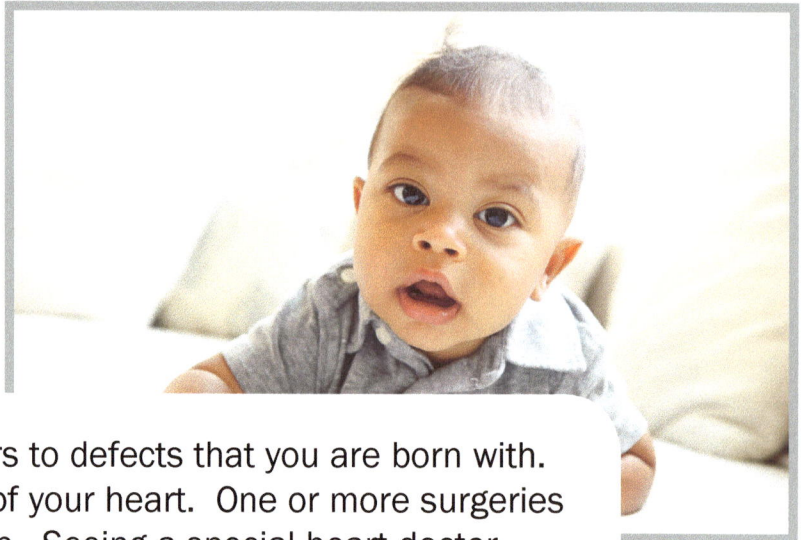

Congenital heart disease refers to defects that you are born with. Often they increase the work of your heart. One or more surgeries to repair the defect(s) can help. Seeing a special heart doctor can help in treating symptoms from high blood pressure, coronary artery or lung disease.

Transposition of the great arteries (TGA)

TGA occurs when the pulmonary artery comes out of the lower left chamber and the aorta comes out of the lower right chamber.

When the aorta and pulmonary artery are reversed, the body doesn't get the oxygen-rich blood that it should. **The right heart** recycles the same blood through the arteries and veins without a way to get more oxygen.

The left side of the heart recycles the same oxygen-rich blood through the lungs. For any of the oxygen-rich blood to get into the aorta and out to the body, there has to be one or more holes between the heart chambers and/or a connecting blood vessel.

For years, TGA was corrected by switching the top 2 heart chambers (atria) with a Mustard or Senning operation. Adults who had either operation as a child can develop heart failure if the thinner right ventricle gets tired of pumping blood against the high pressures in the aorta.

Tetralogy of Fallot (TOF)

TOF refers to 4 heart defects. The aorta opens to both of the lower heart chambers above a large hole called a ventricular septal defect or VSD.

In addition, there is narrowing under or at the pulmonary valve (pulmonary stenosis) and thickening (enlargement) of the right lower chamber.

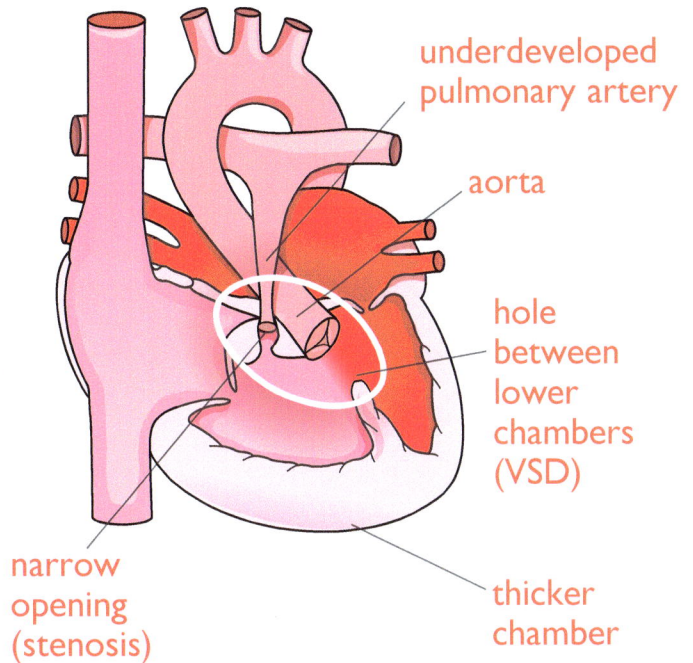

underdeveloped pulmonary artery

aorta

hole between lower chambers (VSD)

narrow opening (stenosis)

thicker chamber

Single ventricle (univentricular heart)

Single ventricle means there is **one ventricle** (lower heart chamber) instead of two separate chambers. This means a large amount of blood is pumped into the lungs. This can damage the blood vessels in the lungs, and the heart valves can also be affected.

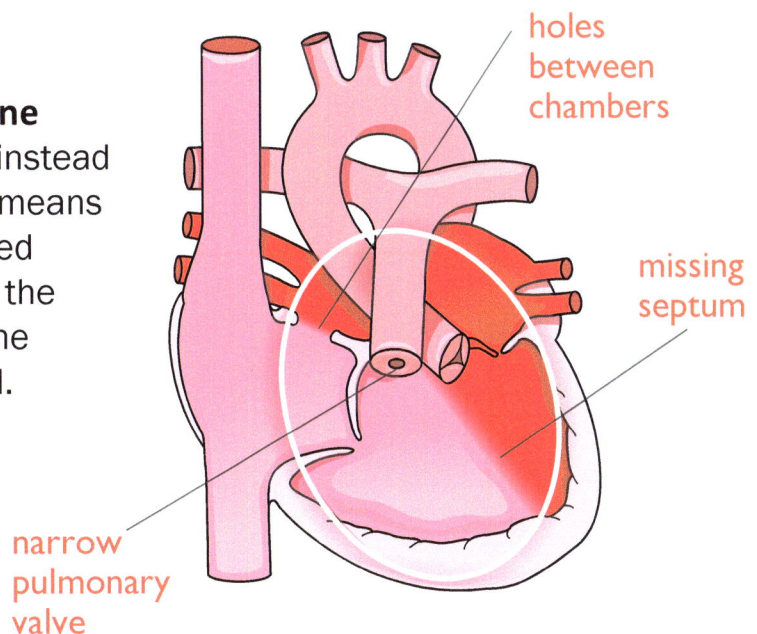

holes between chambers

missing septum

narrow pulmonary valve